FOOD DIGESTION

Food Digestion: Known What You
Eat And How It Digest And Add
The Needed Nutrient To Your
Body For Good Health

Mary f. Phipps

Table of Contents

CHAPTER ONE 3

FOOD DIGESTION 3

How a great deal time it expects
to take in food 3

What happens all through food
absorption 7

This happens when you take in
food: 8

CHAPTER TWO 12

ATTAINABLE

GASTROINTESTINAL

DIFFICULTIES 12

Pointers for better food processing 15

Endeavor these pointers: 16

Limit red meat and refined food varieties 16

Comprise of probiotics for an eating regimen plan 17

Practice everyday 17

Get incredible arrangements of rest 18

Handle endlessly pressure and tension 18

The focus point......................19

CHAPTER THREE......................21

HOW LONG FOOD STAY IN YOUR PAUNCH..........................21

Size of time food stay before leave your obstinate stomach .23

Recreation:..............................24

Food processing:.....................24

Emptying:...............................25

Little gastrointestinal framework:..............................25

Enormous gastrointestinal framework:...........................26

Consistency 27

Calorie articles 28

Sustenance articles 29

Sum 30

CHAPTER FOUR.......................32

INSTRUCTIONS TO BE AWARE ON THE OFF CHANCE THAT YOUR STOMACH IS EMPTY.....32

Safe chance to take medications on void stomach 33

Grapefruit:................................35

Vitamin K: 35

High fat dishes: 35

When to take prescriptions with

food 36

It brings down adverse

consequences: 36

It helps with an issue: 37

It helps with assimilation: 37

When to consume in the event

of treatment 39

The benefits 41

CHAPTER FIVE 44

FOOD VARIETIES SIMPLE TO

PROCESS....................................44

   What to eat for simple food

   processing 45

   Sorts of food easy to absorb....46

   Tinned or prepared natural

   products 47

   Extraordinary choices in this

   food group comprise of:.........47

   Meat things as well as solid and

   adjusted sound protein...........50

Grains 51

Milk things 54

CHAPTER SIX 55

DIFFERENT FOOD VARIETIES 55

Food sources to forestall 57

Natural products......................58

Veggies 59

Aged food sources 61

Meat things as well as sound and adjusted solid protein 62

Grains..................................63

Milk things 64

Different food sources.............65

CHAPTER SEVEN 67

FOOD   ABSORPTION

INCONVENIENCES 67

Steady anomaly.......................68

Food bigotry...........................69

Marks   of   food   narrow

mindedness comprise of:........70

GERD 72

Marks of GERD comprise of:..72

Provocative   stomach   related

framework sickness.................73

There are 2 sort of IBD: 74

Crohn's disease: 74

Ulcerative colitis: 74

Conceivable outrageous issues75

CHAPTER EIGHT 78

HALTING FOOD ABSORPTION

INCONVENIENCES 78

Run of the mill gastrointestinal

issues......................................80

Eat more reliable dishes..........81

Eat more fiber 83

Eat extraordinary arrangements of shower 85

CHAPTER ONE

FOOD DIGESTION

The particular time it thinks about food to encounter the gastrointestinal framework relies upon the sum and kind of food. Factors like sex, metabolic cycle, and an assortment of digestive issues can besides impact the pace of the gastrointestinal treatment.

How a great deal time it expects to take in food

At the same time, food takes 24 to 72 hrs to move with your gastrointestinal framework. The particular time relies upon the sum and kind of food varieties you have eaten.

The cost is moreover according to factors like your sex, metabolic cycle, and whether you have any kind of gastrointestinal issues that can lower or speed up the treatment.

Initially, food trips sensibly rapidly with your gastrointestinal framework. Inside 6 to 8 hrs, the food has separable its means with your difficult midsection, little digestive framework, and large gastrointestinal framework.

At the point when in your enormous gastrointestinal

framework, the to some degree processed results of your recipe can rest for over a day while it's harmed down significantly more.

The regular contrast for transport time is made out of the adhering to: gastric purging (2 to 5 hours), little stomach related framework transport (2 to 6 hours), colonic vehicle (10 to 59 hours), and entire stomach related framework transport (10 to 73 hrs).

Your food assimilation cost is moreover according to what you have eaten. Meat and fish can require as extensive as 2 days to thoroughly taking in. The solid and adjusted sound proteins and fats they have are point by point parts that take much longer for your body to draw in separated.

Similar, veggies and natural products, which are high in fiber, can move with your framework in a ton substantially less when contrasted with a day. As a matter of fact, these high fiber food varieties help your digestive track run all the more really at the same time.

The fastest to take in are refined, magnificent solace food awesome bars. Your body openings with them in a worry of hrs, rapidly leaving you denying once again.

What happens all through food absorption

Food absorption is the treatment where your body issues down food and takes out the supplements your body needs to run. Anything left is a waste thing, which your body disposes of.

Your gastrointestinal framework is comprised of **5 body organs:**

- mouth
- throat
- midsection
- small   digestive framework

- enormous digestive framework

This happens when you take in food:

As you consume, organs in your mouth present spit. This gastrointestinal fluid has compounds that harm down the starches in your food. The outcome is a soft mass considered a bolus that is less complex to consume.

At the point when you eat, the food migrations down your throat the line that interfaces your mouth for a difficult gut. A solid tissue entryway called the diminishing esophageal sphincter opens to allow the food moves into your difficult midsection.

Acids in your obstinate gut harm down the food significantly more. This produces a soft blend of gastric juices and somewhat processed food, called toll. This blend movement on your little gastrointestinal framework.

In your small gastrointestinal framework, your pancreatic and liver incorporate their own digestive juices to the blend.

Pancreatic juices harm down carbs, fats, and sound and adjusted solid proteins. Bile from your gallbladder disintegrates fat. Nutrients, different supplements, and shower move with the wall surface region of your little digestive framework into your circulatory system. The undigested component that stays migrations on your enormous gastrointestinal framework.

The large gastrointestinal framework absorbs any kind of excess splash and remaining supplements from the food. The rest wraps up being strong waste, called stool.

Your rectum stockpiles up till
you're prepared to have a stomach
related framework task.

CHAPTER TWO

ATTAINABLE GASTROINTESTINAL DIFFICULTIES

Specific issues can frustrate food absorption and leave you for certain troublesome horrible effects like indigestion, gas, lopsided poo, or detachment of the entrails.

Indigestion happens when the abatement esophageal sphincter debilitates. This empowers corrosive to help from your obstinate stomach into your throat. The essential pointers and signs and side effect are acid reflux.

Celiac issue includes your body insusceptible framework striking and dangerous your digestion tracts when you eat gluten.

Lopsided crap is considerably less poo when contrasted with ordinary. At the point when you do go, the stool is organization and testing to pass. Lopsided poop trigger pointers like swelling and stomach torment.

Diverticulitis makes small sacks in your digestion tracts. Diverticulitis itself doesn't set off pointers, yet in the event that stool gets implanted the sacks, enlarging and disease can happen. This case is depicted as diverticulitis, and markers comprise of stomach torment, relaxed dung, and occasionally heat.

Fiery stomach related framework issue is made out of Crohn's concern and ulcerative colitis. These issues produce relentless expanding in your digestive organs that can causes boil, torment, and ridiculous detachment of the entrails, weight the board, absence of sustenance, and raise one's aggressive statement of colon disease cells.

Irascible stomach related framework condition causes

bothersome markers like gas, detachment of the guts, and lopsided crap, yet isn't really associated with malignant growth cells or different other extensive digestive sickness.

Lactose prejudice recommends your body doesn't have the protein ought to harm down the sugar in milk things. At the point when you eat milk, you acquire markers like bulging, gas, and detachment of the insides.

Pointers for better food processing

To keep up with food redesigning effectively with your digestive framework and stop issues like detachment of the insides and lopsided poo,

Endeavor these pointers:
Eat more eco-most amiable, natural product, and entire grains

Veggies, organic products, and entire grains are abundant wellsprings of fiber. Fiber helps food move with your digestive framework all the more helpfully and completely.

Limit red meat and refined food varieties
Studies unveil red meat creates synthetics that are associated with heart issue.

Comprise of probiotics for an eating regimen plan

These helpful microorganisms help group out the risky parasites in your digestive framework. You will find them in food varieties like yogurt and kefir, and in supplements.

Practice everyday

Revamping your body safeguards your digestive framework redesigning, too. Strolling after dishes can stop gas and swelling. Practice moreover safeguards your weight in look at, which decreases your message beyond a shadow of a doubt tumors cells and different other illness of the gastrointestinal framework.

Get incredible arrangements of rest

An absence of rest is associated with inordinate weight, which can incorporate to issues with your digestive framework.

Handle endlessly pressure and tension

Extra endlessly stress and tension can intensify gastrointestinal issues like acid reflux and irascible stomach related framework condition. Stress-easing procedures, for example, portrayal and yoga practice exercise can help cool your brain.

The focus point

You might actually not think an incredible arrangement in regards to your digestive framework every day. However you will recognize when it's not working ideally by awkward side effects and signs like gas, swelling, intestinal system abnormality, notwithstanding detachment of the guts.

Appreciate what you eat notwithstanding remain stimulated to keep up with your gastrointestinal framework remodeling proficiently

notwithstanding really feel you are
most noteworthy.

CHAPTER THREE

HOW LONG FOOD STAY IN YOUR PAUNCH

Your stomach framework is vital for helping to gas your body with the supplements it substances from the food varieties you eat.

All through food processing, food that you have devoured exercises with your stomach (GI) framework, where it's continuously harmed down, empowering supplements to be retained.

Every region of your GI framework is customized for an alternate feature of food processing. For conditions, your obstinate paunch utilizes both mechanical notwithstanding compound ways to deal with harm down your food. It thereafter eliminates its parts into your little gastrointestinal framework, where sustenance retention happens.

In spite of the fact that it can differ, there are approximates associating with the ordinary time it contemplates food to disposal with your obstinate midsection notwithstanding different pieces of your GI framework.

We should turn out to be essential for the data of basically how this capabilities notwithstanding for the size of time it takes.

Size of time food stay before leave your obstinate stomach Ordinarily talking, it takes with respect to 2 to 4 hrs for food to end from your difficult gut for a little digestive framework.

The particular measure of time can rely upon different factors, like the beauty care products notwithstanding estimation of your dinner, your chemical agents, notwithstanding your sex. Ladies have the inclination to absorb food all the more dynamically contrasted and men.

The adhering to happens when **food enters your obstinate midsection:**

Recreation: The top part of your obstinate tummy relaxes up in buy to fit the food you have eaten. For this reason your stomach area can look rather extended after a dinner.

Food processing: Your obstinate paunch involves musical pivoting as well as crushing developments (mechanical food processing) alongside difficult stomach corrosive notwithstanding proteins (substance food absorption) to harm down your dinner.

Emptying: The pyloric sphincter empowers little measures of food to pass on your obstinate stomach notwithstanding end into your small digestive framework slowly.

In the wake of leaving your difficult stomach, food exercises with your **digestion tracts:**

Little gastrointestinal framework: In your minuscule digestive framework, food blends in with additional stomach liquids. This is where a large portion of the sustenance ingestion happens. Food can spend between 2 to 6 hrs in your minuscule digestive framework.

Enormous gastrointestinal framework: In your colossal gastrointestinal framework (colon), shower is retained, notwithstanding what is left over from food processing is become stool. The shed things from your food spend around 36 hrs in your tremendous digestive framework.

In complete, it can in the middle of between 2 to 5 days for food to end with your whole GI framework.

Speed at which food can be eliminate from your difficult tummy

Food beauty care products can play a huge obligation in for the size of time it ponders your food to leave your obstinate paunch.

We should investigate some fundamental food-related factors that can influence for the size of time it ponders your obstinate tummy to uninhabited.

Consistency

Fluids typically leave your difficult stomach rapidly. For conditions, after you eat a glass of splash, it's assessed that basically 50% of it will positively be left in your obstinate midsection after 10 mines.

Strong food varieties ordinarily should be harmed down notwithstanding melted extra, which suggests they regularly take much longer to leave your difficult paunch. As a matter of fact, it ordinarily takes in regards to 20 to 50% an hr in the past strong food varieties start to leave your obstinate tummy.

Calorie articles

Notwithstanding consistency, food varieties notwithstanding drinks that have as a matter of fact a limited calorie articles regularly leave your obstinate stomach at a ton speedier cost. More prominent calorie food varieties notwithstanding beverages will unquestionably take much longer.

For conditions, while shower dropped fallen leaves your obstinate stomach at a quick value, a more noteworthy calorie fluid, for example, a glass of natural product juice or a milkshake will surely partition all the more dynamically.

Sustenance articles

Food sources notwithstanding refreshments abundant in starches notwithstanding sound and adjusted solid proteins are harmed down quicker in your difficult gut notwithstanding, along these lines; leave your obstinate paunch faster.

By and by, food sources high in fat notwithstanding fiber spend a much longer measure of time in your difficult gut. That is the reason you could really feel total for much longer when you eat food varieties that are high in fat or fiber.

Sum

The estimation of your feast can affect the cost at which food dropped fallen leaves your obstinate stomach. This appears at forestall genuine for the two fluids notwithstanding solids.

It's memorable fundamental that strong dishes will positively ordinarily have as a matter of fact a slack period in the past obstinate midsection purging beginnings. By the by, bigger dishes uninhabited at a great deal speedier cost contrasted and more modest estimated measured dishes as fast as this slack period has passed.

CHAPTER FOUR

INSTRUCTIONS TO BE AWARE ON THE OFF CHANCE THAT YOUR STOMACH IS EMPTY

Regularly talking, on the off chance that it's been various hrs since you have had really anything to consume, your stomach is in all likelihood unfilled.

Notwithstanding, recollect that the pace of stomach-discharging can vary in light of what you have consumed and different variables. Along these lines, time may not continually be a truly precise mark of an empty stomach.

At the point when your stomach is vacant, you could encounter actual indications of desires. Occurrences of these comprise of:

- stomach snarling or distresses
- wooziness
- shortcoming or instability
- migraine
- touchiness

Safe chance to take medications on void stomach

A few drugs should be dealt with an empty stomach. There are a couple of elements for this.

To start with, dental drugs are taken in into your circulatory system through the cell covering of your GI framework. Along these lines, having really food in your stomach might perhaps sluggish a medication's retention, creation it significantly less viable.

Second, there are a few food sources that can impede the undertaking of explicit sorts of meds. This might potentially increment or reduction the level of a medicine in your framework. This sort of correspondence is known as a food-drug correspondence.

A few occurrences of **food-drug interchanges comprise of:**

Grapefruit: Grapefruit can expand the levels of specific drugs in your blood. Cases comprise of certain terminals and hypertension medications.

Vitamin K: Food varieties high in vitamin K, like spinach, kale, and Brussels sprouts, can diminish the adequacy of the blood more slender warfarin.

High fat dishes: Consuming a high fat dish can bring down levels of esomeprazole, a proton siphon inhibitor, in your circulatory system.

On the off chance that food utilization can possibly influence a medicine, your solution will say to take it on an empty stomach.

An incredible norm to follow for these sorts of meds is to take them either 1 hr prior to consuming or 2 hrs subsequent to consuming.

When to take prescriptions with food

Here and there you may be recommended a medicine that illuminates you to take it with food. There are two or three **elements for this:**

It brings down adverse consequences: A few drugs, like

nonsteroidal mitigating prescriptions (NSAIDs) and corticosteroids, can cause stomach upset when dealt with an empty stomach. Having really food in your stomach can assist with bringing down the opportunity of these adverse consequences.

It helps with an issue: A few wellbeing and health issues, similar to diabetes or indigestion, are impacted by food utilization. For that reason taking prescription for these sorts of issues with food is significant.

It helps with assimilation: In some cases having really food in your GI framework can help with medication assimilation. This turns out as expected for certain sorts of HIV medications.

Assuming that you have really a drug that you want to take with food, expect to organize taking your prescription with your supper time.

Continually adhere to the guidelines on the medicine item bundling, and contact your primary care physician or pharmacologist with any inquiries.

When to consume in the event of treatment

A few sorts of tests or medicines might expect you to quick in advance. At the point when you quick, you are shunning consuming for a characterized amount of time. For example, you could have to **quick previously:**

- a few sorts of blood tests, for example, those for glucose and fatty substances
- strategies including the GI framework or stomach region, like an endoscopy or stomach ultrasound

- testing for food unfavorably susceptible responses or bigotries
- medical procedure that is performed utilizing fundamental sedative

On the off chance that you are not eating, you probably won't can consume anything for 6 to 8 hrs before the test or treatment.

For example, in the event that you are having really a treatment in the early morning, you will triumph ultimately your last total dish the prior night and not consume anything until after your treatment.

There might be extra principles connects with what sorts of refreshments you can have. This frequently includes simply drinking a level of sprinkle all through you're not eating term.

The particular guidelines for food and sprinkle utilization can depend on the test or treatment that is being performed. Continually cautiously keep your PCP's guidelines, and go ahead and questions on the off chance that something isn't clear.

The benefits

After you eat, food generally puts 2 to 4 hrs in your stomach. Be that as it may, this can contrast in view of the sort of food you have devoured, how a ton, and different variables.

Liquids ordinarily leave your stomach rapidly, major areas of strength for while normally take significantly longer. Different other food-related factors that can prompt a significantly longer stomach maintenance time **comprise of:**

- high fat food varieties
- high fiber food varieties
- fatty food sources

Whether your stomach is finished or void can influence focuses like taking prescriptions or not eating before an assessment or treatment.

In these situations, it is continually critical to painstakingly adhere to your PCP's guidelines with respect to food and drink utilization.

CHAPTER FIVE

FOOD VARIETIES SIMPLE TO PROCESS

Food varieties that are not difficult to ingest can help with a few signs and issues. **This might comprise of:**

- brief sickness or heaving
- the runs
- gastroenteritis
- gastroesophageal reflux condition (GERD)
- diverticulitis
- fiery intestinal system condition

Whatever the example, picking the right food sources might be the way to keeping away from potential enacts and feeling significantly improved.

What to eat for simple food processing

- Toast
- White rice
- Bananas
- Fruit purée
- Eggs
- Yams
- Chicken
- Salmon
- Gelatin
- Saltine rolls
- Oat dish

Sorts of food easy to absorb

Food sources that are easy to absorb have the penchant to be brought down in fiber. This is since fiber while a sound and endlessly adjusted region of the eating routine is the area of natural products, veggies, as well as grains that isn't really processed by your body. Along these lines, the fiber goes through your enormous digestive framework too as could set off various worries, from gas to swelling too hard to-pass stool.

Devouring food sources that are brought down in fiber diminishes how much undigested thing also as could limit your markers.

Tinned or prepared natural products

Entire organic products have high measures of fiber, yet cooking them helps harm down the fiber extensively that makes it a great deal significantly less convoluted to absorb. Stripping the skin as well as getting rid of the seeds from veggies and organic product will help decline how much fiber.

Extraordinary choices in this food group comprise of:

- very ready banana
- melon

- honeydew melon

- watermelon

- avocado

- fruit purée

- tinned or prepared natural products without the skin or seeds

While consuming any among the over natural products, consume them in small sums as they are crude too as bigger segment estimations might in any case **cause stomach distress.**

Tinned or prepared veggies

Very much like organic product, entire veggies have actually a reasonable setup of fiber. At the point when they're prepared, the fiber will be somewhat harmed down as well as a great deal considerably less muddled to absorb.

You can set up your veggies in your home or find tinned ranges on the shelf's at your neighborhood supermarket. Potatoes without skin as well as pureed tomatoes are different decisions for low-fiber veggies.

Both organic product as well as veggie squeezes that don't have mash is similarly brought down in fiber.

Extraordinary choices of tinned or prepared scopes of **veggies comprise of:**

- yellow squash without seeds
- spinach
- pumpkin
- beets
- green beans
- carrots

Meat things as well as solid and adjusted sound protein
Critical projects of lean sound and adjusted solid protein like chicken, turkey, as well as fish will generally absorb well. Delicate limits of hamburger or pork as

well as ground meats are different other extraordinary decisions. Veggie lovers could endeavor consolidating eggs, lavish nut margarines, or tofu for comprised of solid and adjusted sound protein.

Essentially the way that you plan meat can in like manner influence basically that it is so easy to absorb. Rather contrasted with searing it, endeavor barbecuing, cooking, food readiness, or poaching.

Grains

You might have truly paid attention to that generous entire

grains are best to consume in your eating routine. On the off chance that you're looking for simple to-process grains, **you should stay with:**

- white or further developed breads or rolls
- normal bagels
- white salute
- white rolls

You can in like manner find low-fiber absolutely dry or prepared grains at the supermarket.

Refined treats that don't have dried out natural products or nuts could be gentle on your framework. Typical pasta or noodles as well as pretzels made with further developed flours in like manner misfortune in this group.

Further developed flours (grains) have truly been customized to wipe out the wheat as well as microorganism, producing them a ton considerably less convoluted to absorb. This is instead of crude flours, which experience a ton significantly less calibrating as well as have more noteworthy fiber. Usually, further developed flours are not suggested in that frame of mind as region of a sound and endlessly adjusted diet routine.

Milk things

On the off chance that you're lactose bigoted, milk could trouble your food absorption or trigger detachment of the entrails. Search for things that are sans lactose or brought down in lactose. In any case, milk is brought down in fiber too as could be easy to absorb for extraordinary arrangements of people. Endeavor polishing off liquor typical milk or eating on cheddar, yogurt, as well as home cheddar. High-fat milk food varieties like gelato are not advantageously absorbable.

CHAPTER SIX

DIFFERENT FOOD VARIETIES

All-normal regular spices as need might arise to be used with treatment in cooking. Entire flavors couldn't absorb well. Ranges that are ground should be alright. Lively food varieties as well as large amounts of stew pepper in food sources could cause stomach uneasiness as well as heartburn.

The sticking to food varieties is in like manner sans risk on a low-fiber or delicate **food varieties diet routine:**

- sugar, honey, jam

- mayonnaise

- mustard

- soy sauce

- oil, spread, margarine

- marshmallows

Diminishing any kind of food you eat into small things as well as biting each assault well in the past ingesting can moreover help with food absorption. Make a significant stretch of time for your dishes so you generally aren't consuming rapidly.

While consuming an eating routine that is brought down in fiber, you could see that your specific dung are more modest measured estimated as well as your poo are a ton substantially less consistent. Guarantee you eat incredible arrangements of liquids like splash as well as regular tea over the course of the day to forestall inconsistency.

Food sources to forestall
High-fiber food sources misfortune past of the reach: Notwithstanding fiber, explicit cooking draws near, such as broiling, may trouble your belly. Carbonation as well as high levels of elevated degrees of caffeine, notwithstanding incredibly fiery

food varieties, could set off worries too.

Right recorded underneath are a few food varieties to forestall since they couldn't be easy to absorb.

Natural products

A lot of new natural products have a significant measure of fiber, particularly on the off chance that they have actually the skins or seeds. Conditions of natural products that are a ton considerably less confounded to absorb comprise of bananas as well as avocados. **Organic products to forestall comprise of:**

- dried out natural products
- tinned natural product liquor
- pineapple
- coconut
- frigid or new berries

Keep up with a long way from a natural product or veggie juices which comprise of mash. Tomatoes too as citrus organic products could set off worries particularly for people with GERD.

Veggies

Crude veggies should be safeguarded against as they have significantly more intact fiber contrasted and prepared or tinned. Moreover, you could **wish to forestall:**

- mushrooms
- pan sear veggies
- stewed tomatoes
- potato skins
- dried out beans
- peas
- vegetables
- broccoli
- cauliflower
- onion
- cabbage
- brussels sprouts
- peppers

Aged food sources

Numerous people could wish to keep away from sauerkraut, kamahi, as well as pickles too. In the event that these matured food sources don't trouble you, they truly do have actually the planned to give assistance food processing. This is since some brand name names or homemade variations of these food varieties have "wonderful" microorganisms like probiotics as well as pragmatic food absorption catalysts. These accommodating microorganisms predigest food as well as help you better soak up the supplements.

Review labels steadily on business things to make sure the food truly do have probiotics as well as different other valuable microorganisms as well as doesn't have excessively a great deal comprised of salt or sugar.

Meat things as well as sound and adjusted solid protein

Any sort of meats that are hard or unrefined could be challenging to absorb. These comprise of:

- meats with genuine domains, like franks, hotdog, as well as kielbasa
- lunch meats

- meats with entire preferences
- shellfish

Beans, thick peanut butter, as well as entire nuts are different other sound and adjusted solid protein sources that could give you some issue going through your stomach framework.

Grains

The greater part of tweaked grains is advantageously absorbable. That proposes that entire grain breads, rolls, as well as bagels are not continually extraordinary choices.

Keep an eye out for grain things which comprise of raisins, nuts, as well as seeds, for example, multigrain bread rolls. Besides stay liberated from oats which comprise of nuts, dried out organic products, as well as grain.

Granola, brown or wild rice, also as entire grain pasta couldn't absorb advantageously by the same token.

Milk things

While individuals who are lactose prejudiced could plan to remain free from the vast majority of milk things, they could endure yogurt or kefir. The sound and endlessly adjusted microorganisms in these food varieties help to harm down the lactose sugar, fabricating them easier to take in.

You can make your own yogurt or searching for ranges that especially have probiotics.

Moreover, remain liberated from any sort of milk things that are joined with new natural product, seeds, nuts, or made sugars.

Different food sources
Different food sources you might actually expect to remain liberated from comprise of:

- jams as well as jams which incorporate seeds, treats, as well as entire preferences

- carbonated drinks (like pop)

- energized drinks (like espresso)

- liquor

- hot or rotisserie food sources (could give you acid reflux or heartburn)

CHAPTER SEVEN

FOOD ABSORPTION INCONVENIENCES

The gastrointestinal framework is a top to bottom as well as broad component of the body. It contrasts absolutely from the mouth to the rectum. The digestive framework helps your body ingest critical supplements as well as is liable for disposing of shed.

Food absorption issues can show above negative markers. Little issues that are left disregarded can create more limit, tireless problems.

Because of that there are a ton of different sort of food processing issues, you could erroneously deny them. It's fundamental to grasp commonplace food processing issues along with crisis circumstance situation pointers so you distinguish when to chat with a specialist.

Steady anomaly

Steady inconsistency shows an issue with disposing of sheds. This typically happens when the colon can't pass or move defecation through the remainder of the gastrointestinal framework. You might actually encounter stomach torment as well as swelling along with substantially less crap (which are more anguishing when contrasted with typical).

Tenacious anomaly is just among one of quite possibly of the most average gastrointestinal issue in the Consolidated adequate fiber, splash, as well as exercise will positively without a doubt help diminish anomaly. Prescriptions can besides offer mitigation in additional outrageous conditions.

Food bigotry

Food bigotry happens when your digestive framework can't endure specific food varieties. Not at all like food sensitivities, which can set off hives as well as slowly inhaling issues, has a prejudice just effected food processing.

Marks of food narrow mindedness comprise of:

- bulging as well as/or throbs
- detachment of the guts
- headache
- indigestion
- fretfulness
- gas
- hurling

Food narrow mindedness not entirely settled by saving as well as surveying a food journal. Recording what you eat when will assist you with figuring out which food varieties are setting off your markers.

Celiac disease, an immune system issue, is one sort of food narrow mindedness. It creates gastrointestinal issues when you eat gluten (a sound and adjusted solid protein in wheat, grain, as well as rye). Individuals with celiac sickness need to stick to a sans gluten diet intend to diminish pointers as well as issues to the minuscule gastrointestinal framework.

GERD

Indigestion is an ordinary event for a few adults. This happens when obstinate tummy acids go help into the throat, setting off bust torment as well as the trademark defrosting experience.

On the off chance that you have very more predictable indigestion, you could have gastro esophageal reflux illness (GERD). Such reliable episodes can forestall your day to day live as well as issues your throat.

Marks of GERD comprise of:
- bosom distress
- totally dry hacking

- harsh decision in the mouth
- hurting throat
- ingesting issues

You might actually expect meds to control acid reflux. A harmed throat can make ingesting testing as well as disturb the remainder of the digestive framework.

Provocative stomach related framework sickness

Provocative stomach related framework infirmity (IBD) is a kind of industrious enlarging. It influences among additional pieces of the digestive framework.

There are 2 sort of IBD:

Crohn's disease: influences the whole digestive (GI) framework at this point a large portion of regularly influences the minuscule gastrointestinal framework as well as the colon

Ulcerative colitis: influences just the colon IBD can set off additional essential gastrointestinal issues, for example, stomach torment as well as detachment of the insides. **Different pointers can comprise of:**

- depletion
- inadequate poo

- anorexia nervosa as well as flourishing weight reduction
- evening sweats
- butt-centric discharging

It's fundamental for clinical analysis as well as manages IBD in a split second. Not just will unquestionably you be more agreeable, yet extremely early treatment moreover diminishes issues to the GI framework.

Conceivable outrageous issues

A gastroenterologist is a specialist that focuses on perceiving as well as dealing with illness comprising of the digestive framework. In the event that you stay to encounter food processing issues, it's time creation a visit.

A few signs are more limits too as can demonstrate there's a crisis circumstance situation clinical trouble. **These signs comprise of:**

- ridiculous defecation
- consistent throwing up
- outrageous stomach hurts
- perspiring
- sudden, surprising weight the executives

These markers can be a sign of a disease, gallstones, hepatitis, inside discharging, or malignant growth cells.

CHAPTER EIGHT

HALTING FOOD ABSORPTION INCONVENIENCES

The gastrointestinal framework is important to assisting your body with harming down food to guarantee that it can without a doubt satisfactorily recover supplements as well as nutrients while similarly disposing of shed. It's included the **adhering to body organs:**

- mouth
- throat
- liver
- stomach
- gallbladder

- little as well as colossal digestion tracts
- pancreatic
- butt as well as rectum

When something is intruded on inside the digestive framework, you could encounter undesirable markers.

A few issues are significant adequate to require a look at to a gastroenterologist, an expert that arrangement with gastrointestinal worries. Others are basically partners to way of life regimens.

Run of the mill gastrointestinal issues

Among perhaps of the most regular gastrointestinal issue comprise of:

- abnormality
- detachment of the entrails
- gas
- indigestion (heartburn)
- sickness or hurling as well as throwing up
- stomach related throbs

Keep up with analyzing to find a few of among perhaps of the most believed strategy you can without a doubt help stop regular food processing issues, as well as ways of recognizing when to phone telephone discussion the clinical expert.

Eat more reliable dishes
Incredible arrangements of weight the executives' ally consuming more modest measured estimated, more reliable dishes to help work on metabolic rate as well as keep up with you from over-eating. This standard jars without a doubt moreover help stop food processing issues.

At the point when you eat an enormous feast, your digestive framework is over-burden as well as it probably won't have the ability to manage food along with it ought to. This can without a doubt foster indigestion from acids getting back from the belly into the throat. Such stomach over-burden could likewise cause gas, nausea or hurling, or throwing up.

Significance to ingest 5 to 6 small feasts a day can without a doubt help market essential great digestive wellbeing and wellbeing. Ensure you eat a blend of carbs, sound and adjusted solid protein, as well as heart-sound fat at every feast. Conditions comprise of peanut butter on entire wheat bread rolls, a fish sandwich, or yogurt with natural product.

You ought to in like manner stay liberated from present down subsequent to consuming. This lifts the gamble of indigestion as well as nausea or hurling.

Eat more fiber

You could have paid attention to an enormous sum viewing fiber for weight the board as well as heart health and wellbeing. At the point when it alludes to gastrointestinal wellbeing and wellbeing, fiber is similarly a significant viewpoint.

Fiber is the mass in extend food sources that can't be processed.

Solvent fiber makes a gel in the gastrointestinal framework to keep up with you complete, while insoluble fiber comprises of mass to excrement.

The Mayo Place suggests an all-out amount day to day fiber utilization of 38 grams for individuals under 50, as well as 25 grams for women in the specific identical age. Adults north of 50 require somewhat a ton substantially less fiber, with 30 grams per day for individuals as well as 21 grams for women.

Gaining adequate fiber helps stop food absorption issues by dealing with the framework. Assuming you're dubious in the event that you get adequate fiber, you should simply peruse in your kitchen region area. Fiber is ordinarily **promptly accessible in:**

- organic products
- veggies
- beans
- vegetables
- whole grains

Eat extraordinary arrangements of shower

Shower helps your gastrointestinal wellbeing and wellbeing by helping to clean the whole framework. It's especially reasonable in quitting abnormality since shower helps relax your excrement. Moreover, splash could help your gastrointestinal framework retains supplement better by helping the body to harm down food.

Objective to eat 8 glasses of shower a day as well as stay away from the wonderful beverages. Comprised of sugars can without a doubt make food processing issues likewise much more dreadful.

At the point when digestive worries require a specialist's probably going to

At the point when food processing issues can't settle with calibrates in your way of life, it very well may be an ideal opportunity to schedule an evaluation with a gastroenterologist. Constant (reoccurring) issues can show wellbeing and wellbeing worries that could require clinical pace of enthusiasm. **These could comprise of:**

- indigestion
- celiac issue
- colitis
- Crohn's concern
- ulcerative colitis
- gallstones
- grouchy stomach related framework condition (IBS)

- outrageous viral or parasitical contaminations

These worries can't be tended to without clinical pace of enthusiasm.

You ought to see a specialist right away on the off chance that you experience extreme stomach torment, ridiculous defecation, or unforeseen weight the board.

www.ingramcontent.com/pod-product-compliance
Lightning Source LLC
Chambersburg PA
CBHW051827250726
48659CB00005B/1710